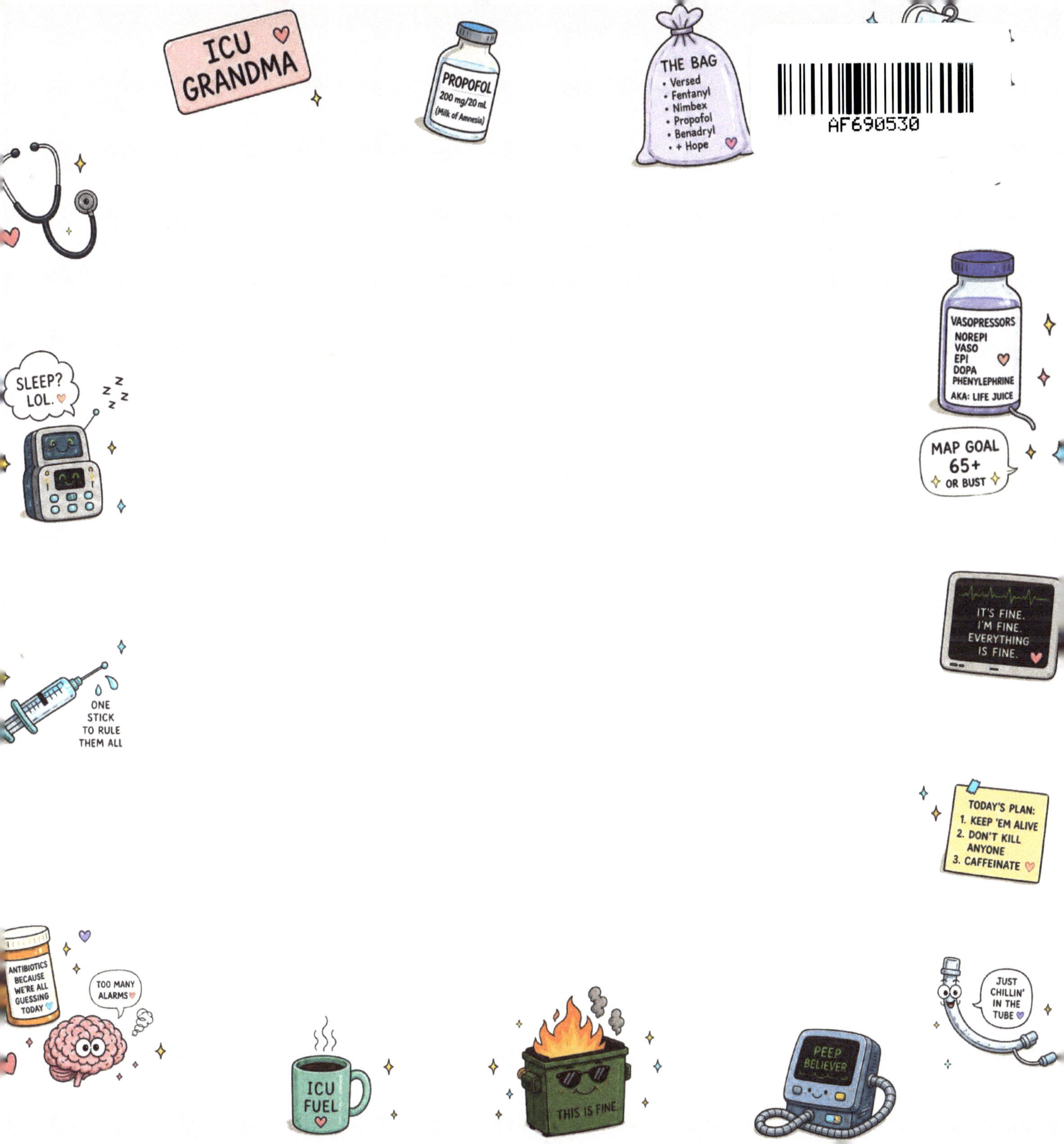
ICU GRANDMA
PROPOFOL
200 mg/20 mL
(Milk of Amnesia)
THE BAG
• Versed
• Fentanyl
• Nimbex
• Propofol
• Benadryl
• + Hope
SLEEP? LOL.
VASOPRESSORS
NOREPI
VASO
EPI
DOPA
PHENYLEPHRINE
AKA: LIFE JUICE
MAP GOAL 65+ OR BUST
IT'S FINE. I'M FINE. EVERYTHING IS FINE.
ONE STICK TO RULE THEM ALL
TODAY'S PLAN:
1. KEEP 'EM ALIVE
2. DON'T KILL ANYONE
3. CAFFEINATE
ANTIBIOTICS BECAUSE WE'RE ALL GUESSING TODAY
TOO MANY ALARMS
JUST CHILLIN' IN THE TUBE
ICU FUEL
THIS IS FINE.
PEEP BELIEVER

AF690530

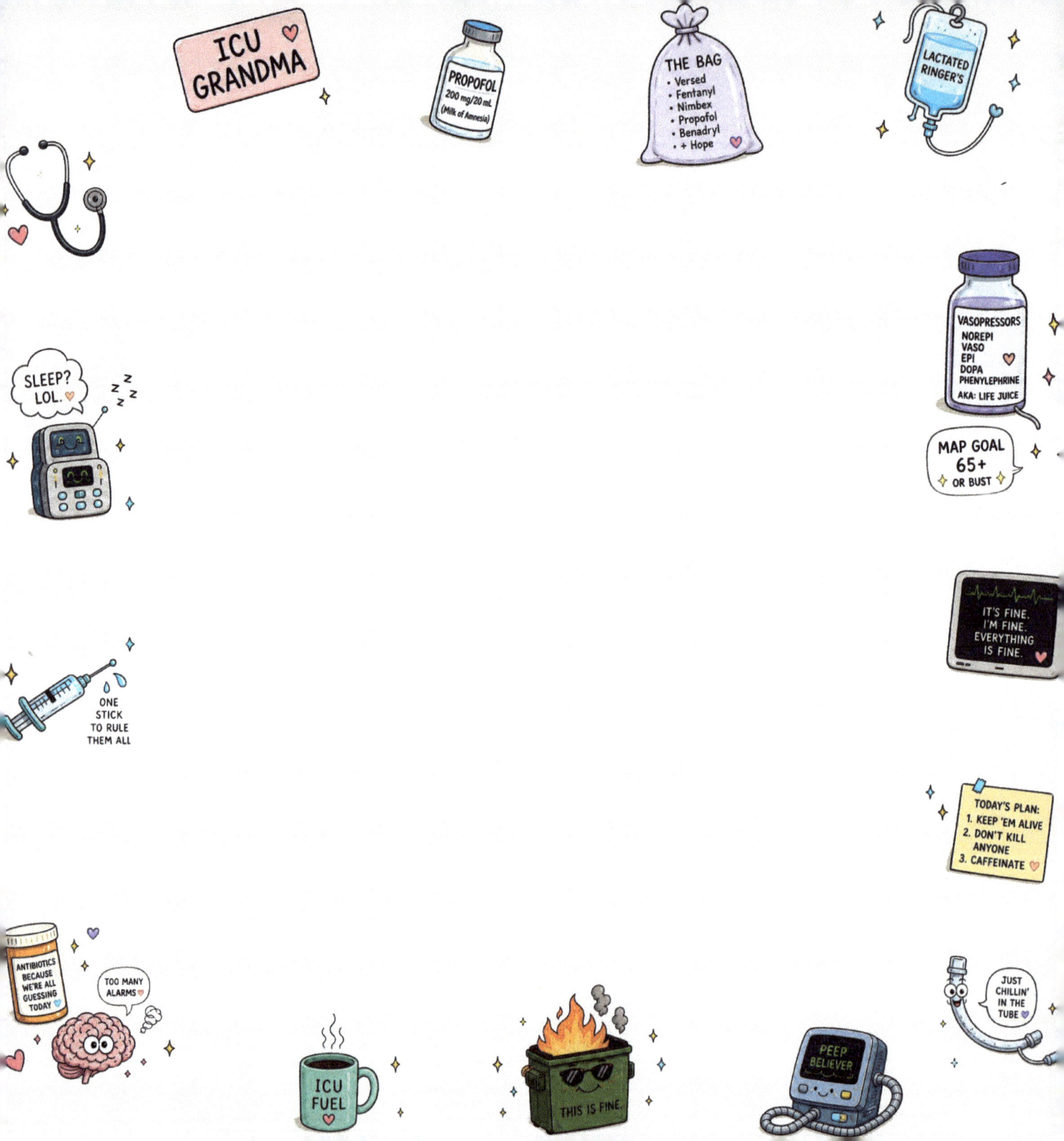
ICU GRANDMA
PROPOFOL 200 mg/20 mL (Milk of Amnesia)
THE BAG
• Versed
• Fentanyl
• Nimbex
• Propofol
• Benadryl
• + Hope
LACTATED RINGER'S
VASOPRESSORS
NOREPI
VASO
EPI
DOPA
PHENYLEPHRINE
AKA: LIFE JUICE
MAP GOAL 65+ OR BUST
SLEEP? LOL.
IT'S FINE. I'M FINE. EVERYTHING IS FINE.
ONE STICK TO RULE THEM ALL
TODAY'S PLAN:
1. KEEP 'EM ALIVE
2. DON'T KILL ANYONE
3. CAFFEINATE
ANTIBIOTICS BECAUSE WE'RE ALL GUESSING TODAY
TOO MANY ALARMS
JUST CHILLIN' IN THE TUBE
ICU FUEL
THIS IS FINE.
PEEP BELIEVER

ICU Grandma

Written by Lee Daniels

Illustrations: by Wolfordeer Colony studio

Published by Griffin Intellectual Property, LLC.

Background graphics by kjpargeter on Mgnific.com

Ebook ISBN: 979-8-9959079-0-9

Paperback ISBN: 979-8-9959079-1-6

Hardback ISBN: 979-8-9959079-2-3

Authors Note

This book is not a children's story.

It uses the language and format of a picture book to tell an adult story about illness. It is intended for mature readers and may be emotionally difficult for some.

All characters and events are fictionalized.

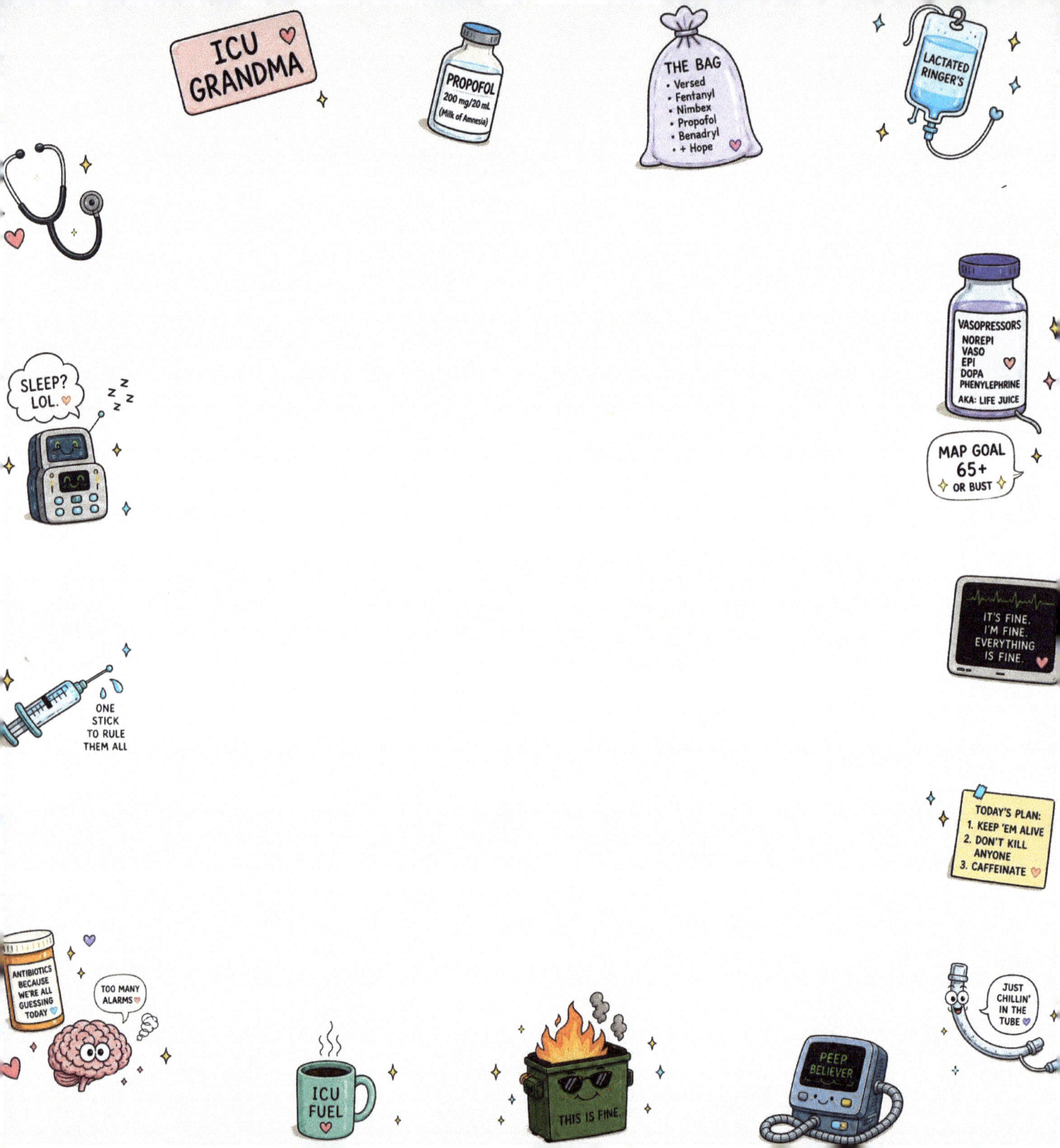
ICU GRANDMA
PROPOFOL 200 mg/20 mL (Milk of Amnesia)
THE BAG
• Versed
• Fentanyl
• Nimbex
• Propofol
• Benadryl
• + Hope
LACTATED RINGER'S
SLEEP? LOL.
VASOPRESSORS
NOREPI
VASO
EPI
DOPA
PHENYLEPHRINE
AKA: LIFE JUICE
MAP GOAL 65+ OR BUST
IT'S FINE. I'M FINE. EVERYTHING IS FINE.
ONE STICK TO RULE THEM ALL
TODAY'S PLAN:
1. KEEP 'EM ALIVE
2. DON'T KILL ANYONE
3. CAFFEINATE
ANTIBIOTICS BECAUSE WE'RE ALL GUESSING TODAY
TOO MANY ALARMS
ICU FUEL
THIS IS FINE.
PEEP BELIEVER
JUST CHILLIN' IN THE TUBE

Dedication

This book is dedicated to Grandma.

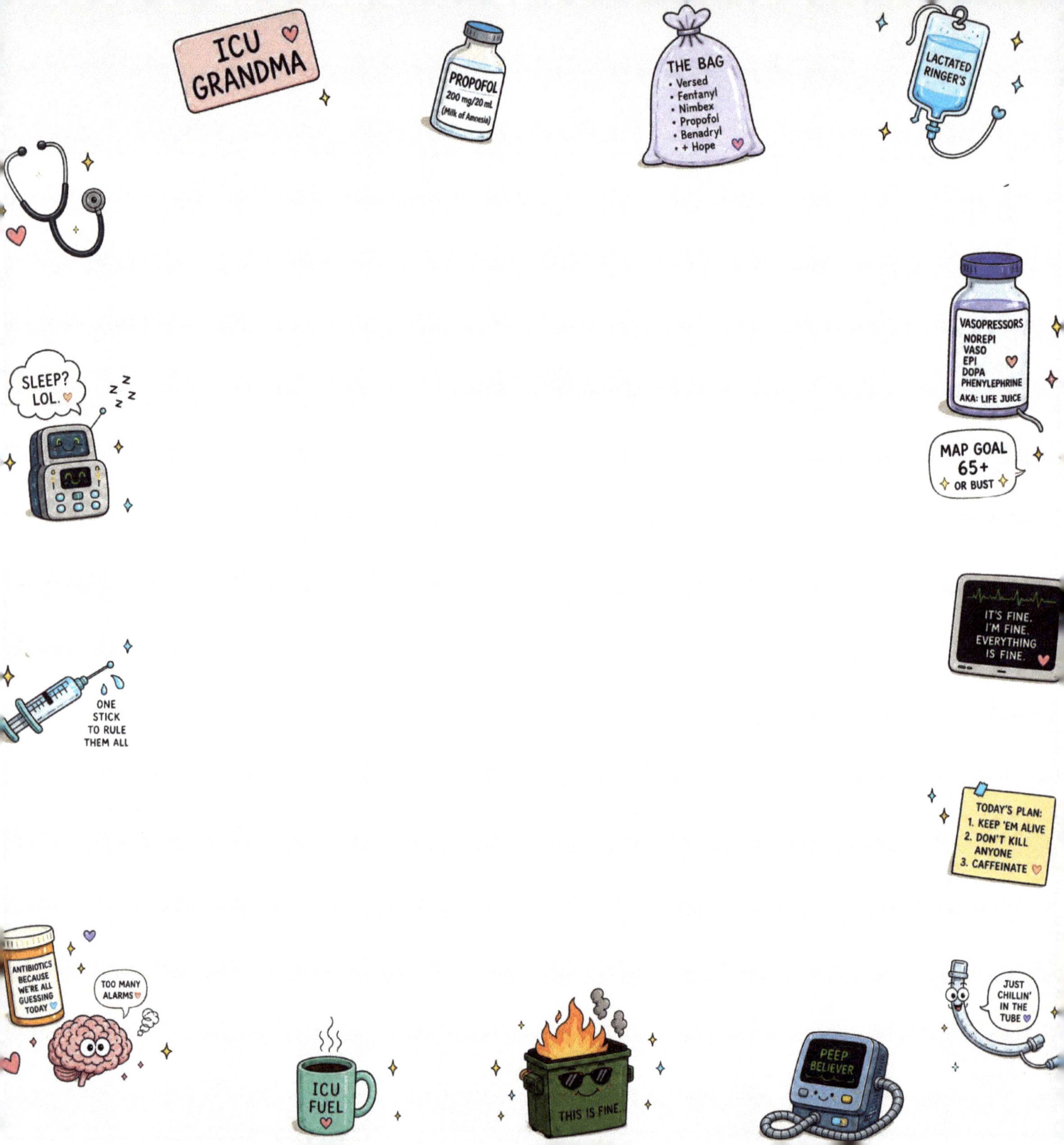
ICU GRANDMA
PROPOFOL
200 mg/20 mL
(Milk of Amnesia)
THE BAG
• Versed
• Fentanyl
• Nimbex
• Propofol
• Benadryl
• + Hope
LACTATED RINGER'S
SLEEP? LOL.
Z Z Z Z
VASOPRESSORS
NOREPI
VASO
EPI
DOPA
PHENYLEPHRINE
AKA: LIFE JUICE
MAP GOAL 65+ OR BUST
IT'S FINE. I'M FINE. EVERYTHING IS FINE.
ONE STICK TO RULE THEM ALL
TODAY'S PLAN:
1. KEEP 'EM ALIVE
2. DON'T KILL ANYONE
3. CAFFEINATE
ANTIBIOTICS BECAUSE WE'RE ALL GUESSING TODAY
TOO MANY ALARMS
JUST CHILLIN' IN THE TUBE
ICU FUEL
THIS IS FINE.
PEEP BELIEVER

Grandma, Grandma, I see you there.

There are bright lights outside.
Mom and Dad are talking very fast.
A man is helping carry you away.
They say you have to go to the hospital now.
They say you are very sick.

I do not know what is wrong.
Everyone is moving fast.
I hope they can make you better.

I see you, Grandma.

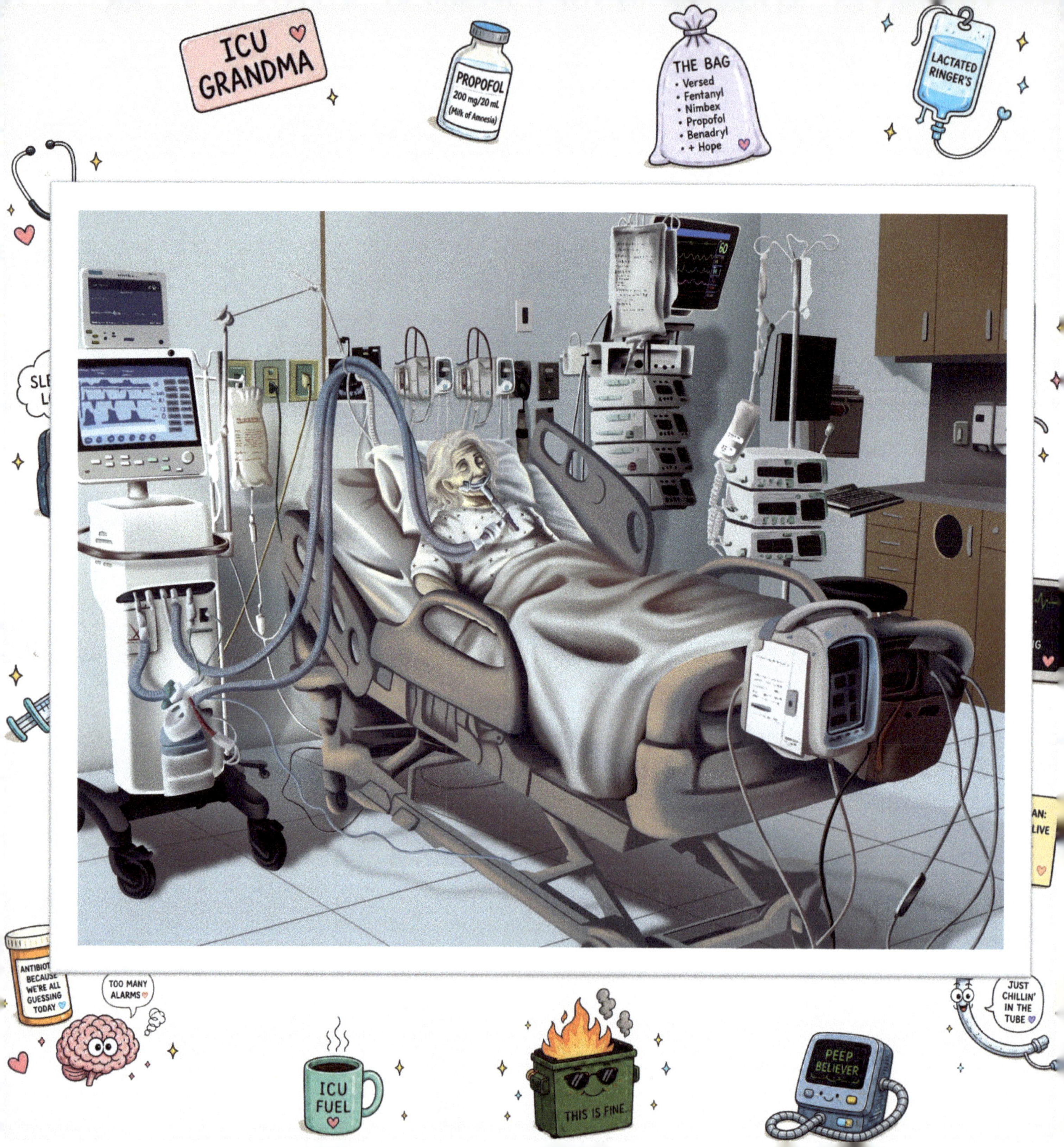
ICU GRANDMA
PROPOFOL
200 mg/20 mL
(Milk of Amnesia)
THE BAG
• Versed
• Fentanyl
• Nimbex
• Propofol
• Benadryl
• + Hope
LACTATED RINGER'S
BECAUSE WE'RE ALL GUESSING TODAY
TOO MANY ALARMS
ICU FUEL
THIS IS FINE.
PEEP BELIEVER
JUST CHILLIN' IN THE TUBE

Grandma, Grandma, I see you there.
You are in your bed.
You look like you are resting so peacefully.
Mom and Dad are talking to the doctors.
They say you are not doing well.
But you look so good and clean.

Usually when we visit, you do not know who I am.
You yell a lot.
Sometimes you are covered in food and smell like pee.
At least now you look nice.

Mom and Dad say the doctors are going to do everything they can to keep you alive.
I am glad.
I hope all this extra medicine will make you better.
Maybe one day you will remember who I am again.
I see you, Grandma.

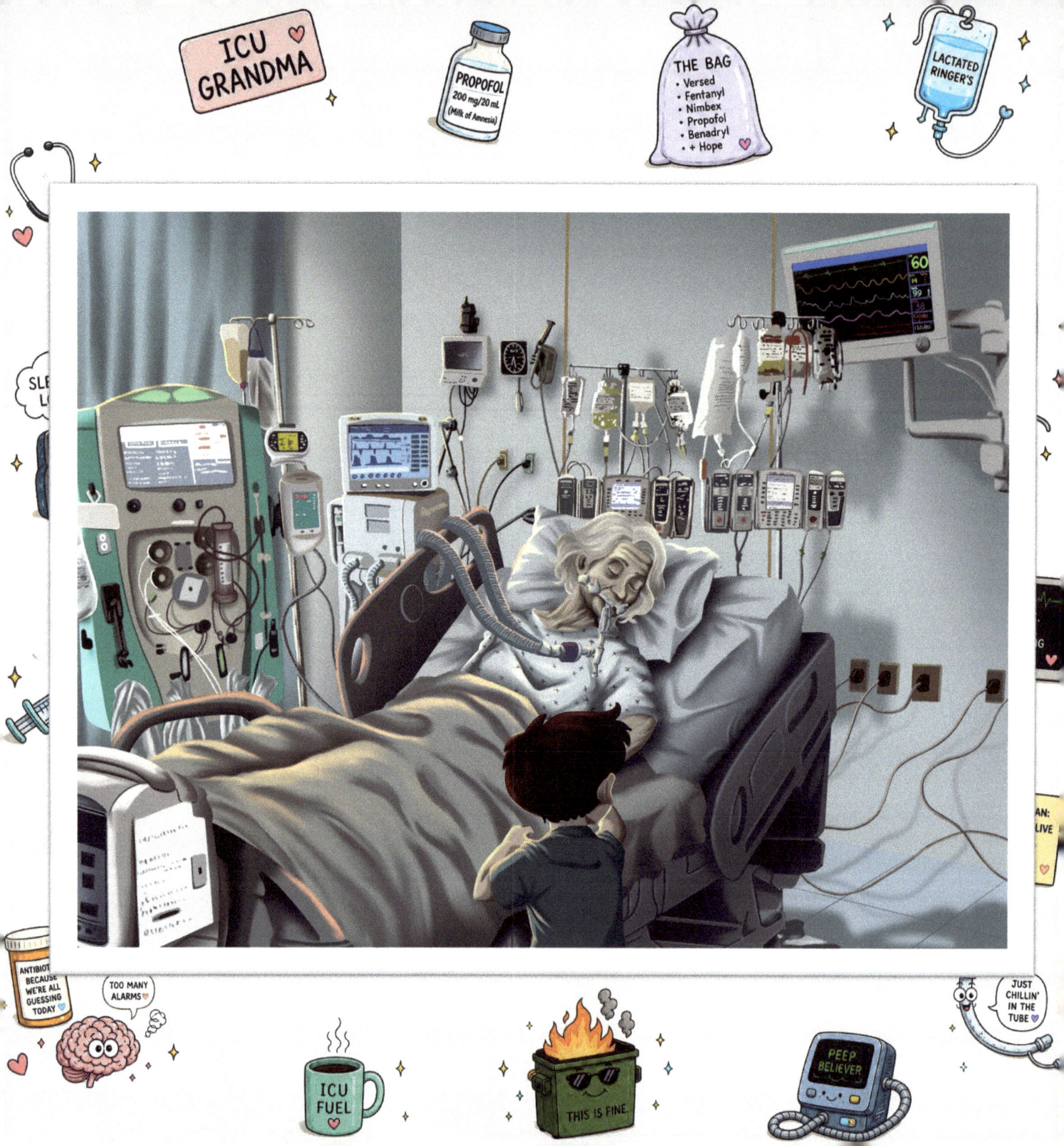
ICU GRANDMA
PROPOFOL
200 mg/20 mL
(Milk of Amnesia)
THE BAG
• Versed
• Fentanyl
• Nimbex
• Propofol
• Benadryl
• + Hope
LACTATED RINGER'S
BECAUSE WE'RE ALL GUESSING TODAY
TOO MANY ALARMS
ICU FUEL
THIS IS FINE.
PEEP BELIEVER
JUST CHILLIN' IN THE TUBE

Grandma, Grandma, I see you there.
You are still in the same bed.
It has been several days now.

The doctors say you have not gotten better.
There are more machines in your room now.

You still look peaceful.
It looks like someone washed your hair.

The doctors are worried you may not make it through the night.
Mom and Dad say they want you to have the very best care.

I see you, Grandma.

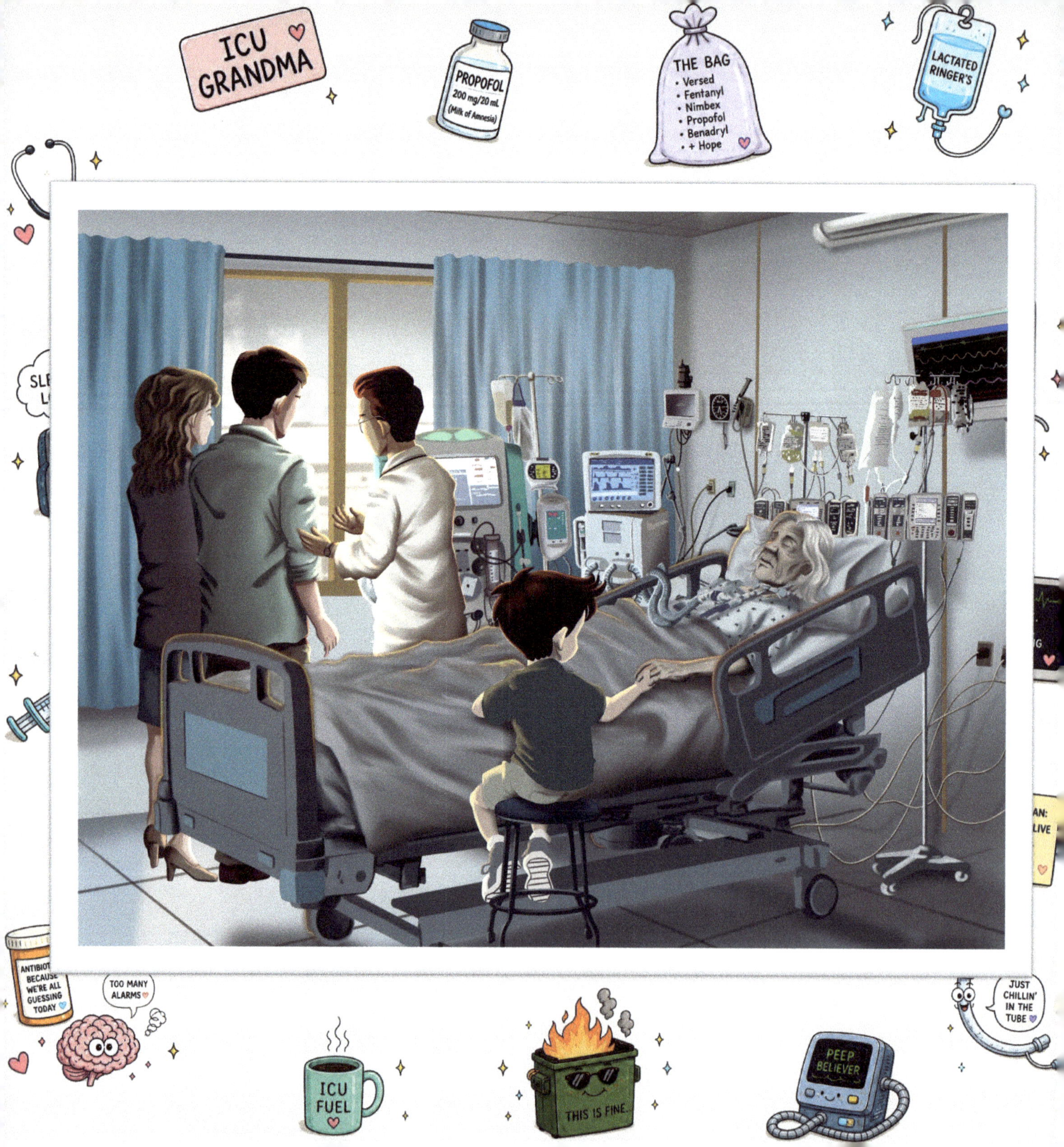
ICU GRANDMA
PROPOFOL 200 mg/20 mL (Milk of Amnesia)
THE BAG
• Versed
• Fentanyl
• Nimbex
• Propofol
• Benadryl
• + Hope
LACTATED RINGER'S
WE'RE ALL GUESSING TODAY
TOO MANY ALARMS
ICU FUEL
THIS IS FINE
PEEP BELIEVER
JUST CHILLIN' IN THE TUBE

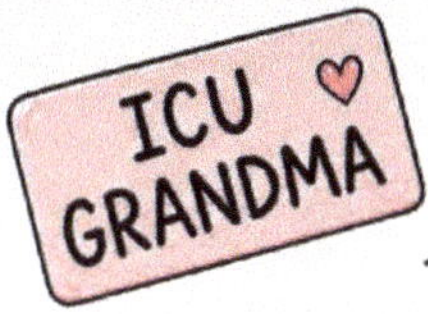

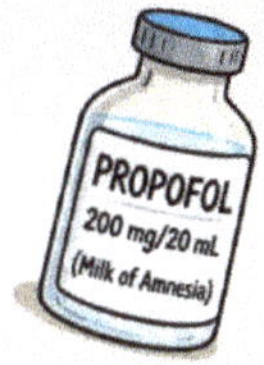

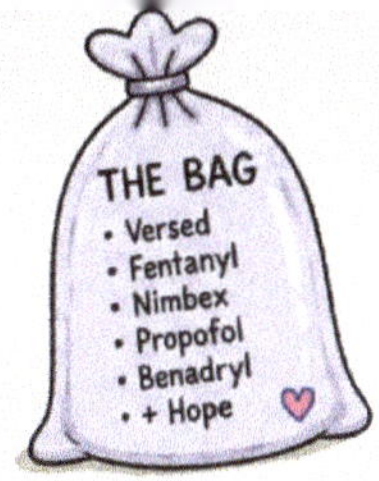

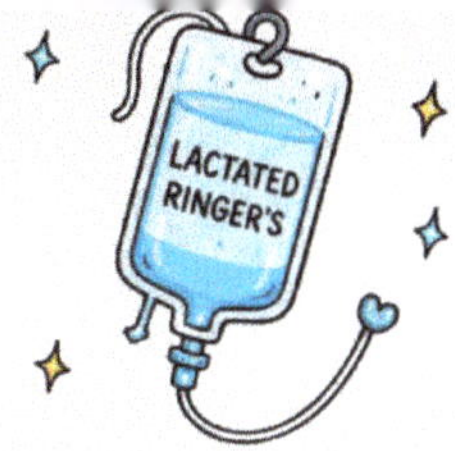

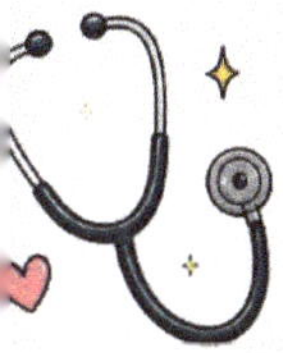

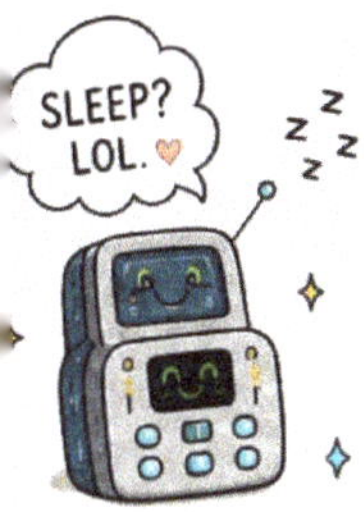

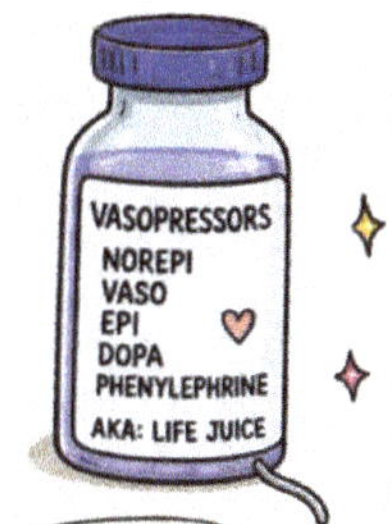

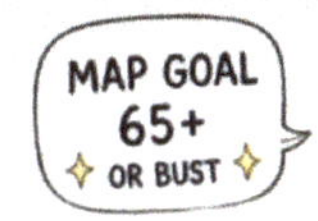

Grandma, Grandma, I see you there.
You are still in your bed.
You made it through the night.
The doctors say things are a little better.

They want to take the tube out of your mouth
and put one in the front of your neck.
They also want to put in a tube for food.
Mom and Dad want this done soon.

After that, they say you will go to another hospital
so you can get stronger.
You have not been out of bed in weeks now,
so I know you need this.
Maybe you can come home again soon.

I see you, Grandma.

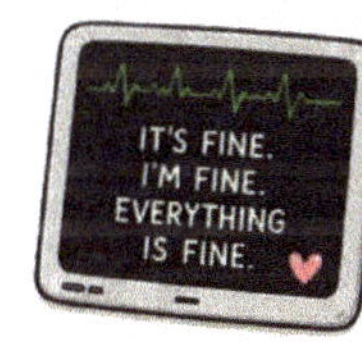

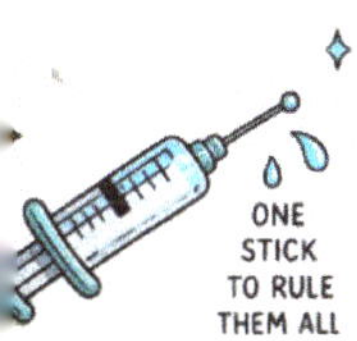

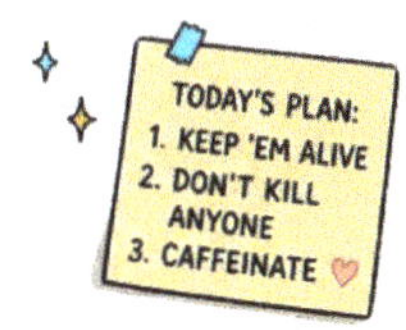

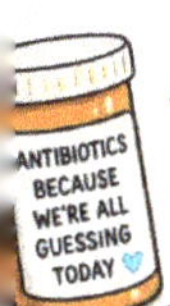

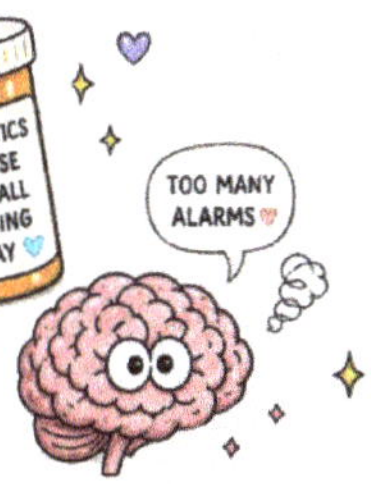

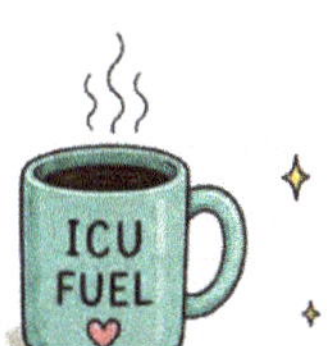

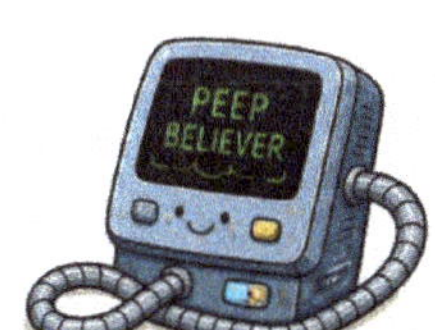

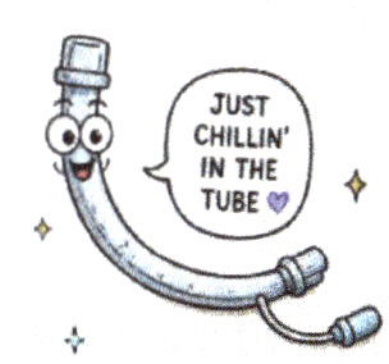

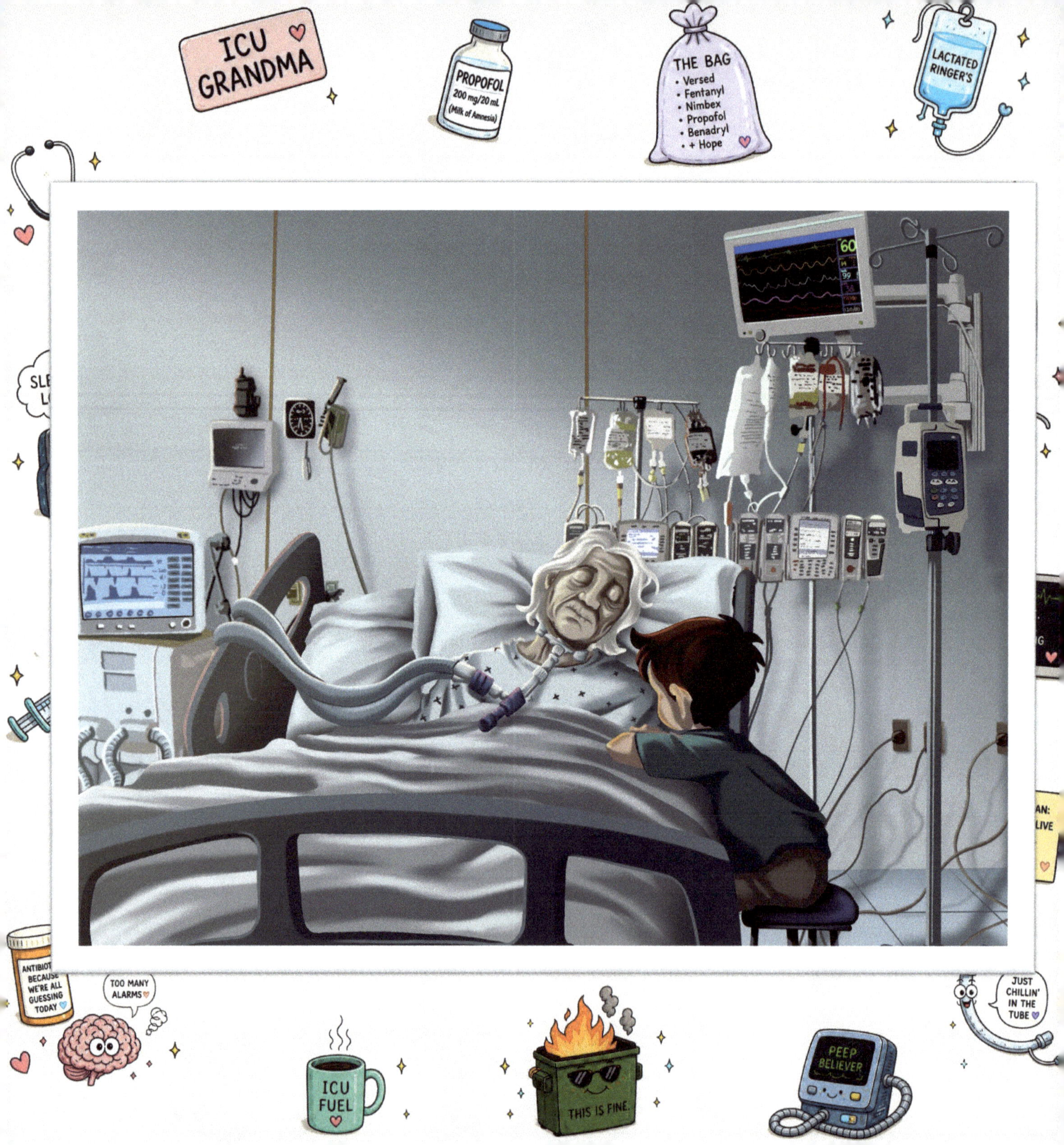
ICU GRANDMA
PROPOFOL
200 mg/20 mL
(Milk of Amnesia)
THE BAG
• Versed
• Fentanyl
• Nimbex
• Propofol
• Benadryl
• + Hope
LACTATED RINGER'S
TOO MANY ALARMS
ICU FUEL
THIS IS FINE.
PEEP BELIEVER
JUST CHILLIN' IN THE TUBE

Grandma, Grandma, I see you there.
You are in a new hospital now.
Your eyes are open, but you are not talking.
You do not move very much.

They feed you through the tube.
You still need the machine to breathe for you.

I do not think you remember me.
Before, you could at least talk.
I hope you can talk to me again soon.
Even if you do not remember who I am.

I see you, Grandma.

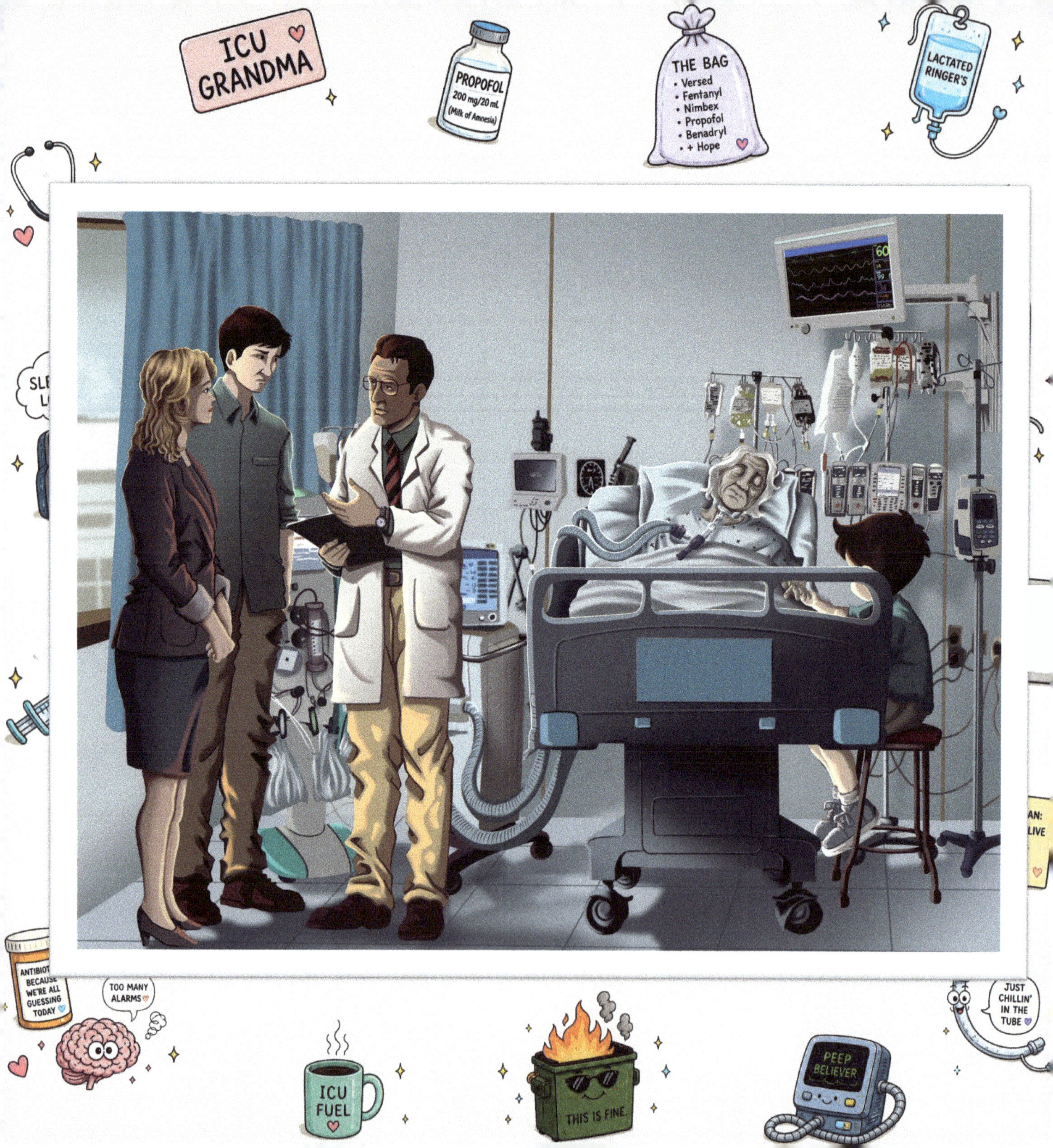
ICU GRANDMA
PROPOFOL
200 mg/20 mL
(Milk of Amnesia)
THE BAG
• Versed
• Fentanyl
• Nimbex
• Propofol
• Benadryl
• + Hope
LACTATED RINGER'S
ANTIBIOT
BECAUSE
WE'RE ALL
GUESSING
TODAY
TOO MANY ALARMS
ICU FUEL
THIS IS FINE.
PEEP BELIEVER
JUST CHILLIN' IN THE TUBE

Grandma, Grandma, I see you there.
It has been over a month now
since you first went to the hospital.
You are still in bed all day.
You still cannot eat or speak.

The doctors say this is your new "normal."
I do not know what that means.

I thought you would be better by now.
I do not understand.
They did so much to help you.

But you are still not better.

Mom and Dad say they are making sure
you get the best care.
They are worried you are getting sick again.

I see you, Grandma.

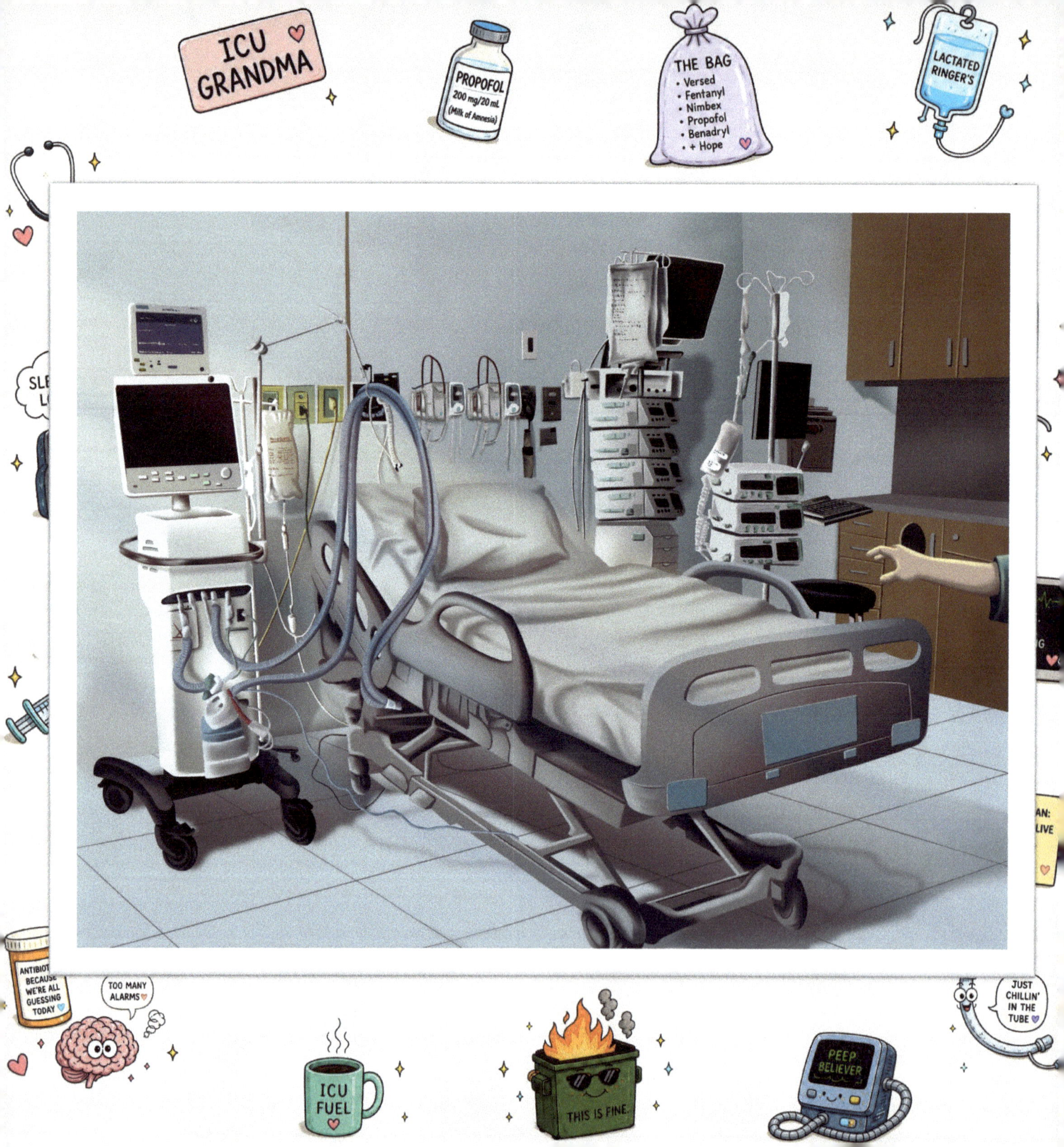

ICU GRANDMA
PROPOFOL 200 mg/20 mL (Milk of Amnesia)
THE BAG
• Versed
• Fentanyl
• Nimbex
• Propofol
• Benadryl
• + Hope
LACTATED RINGER'S
TOO MANY ALARMS
WE'RE ALL GUESSING TODAY
ICU FUEL
THIS IS FINE.
PEEP BELIEVER
JUST CHILLIN' IN THE TUBE

Grandma, Grandma, I see you there.
You had to go back to the hospital.
You did not have a good night.

Mom and Dad tell me you died.
I am very sad.

You spent a long time in the hospital,
but you did not get better.
I hoped you would come home again.
I hoped you would remember me.

I did not get to tell you goodbye.
But I saw you, Grandma.

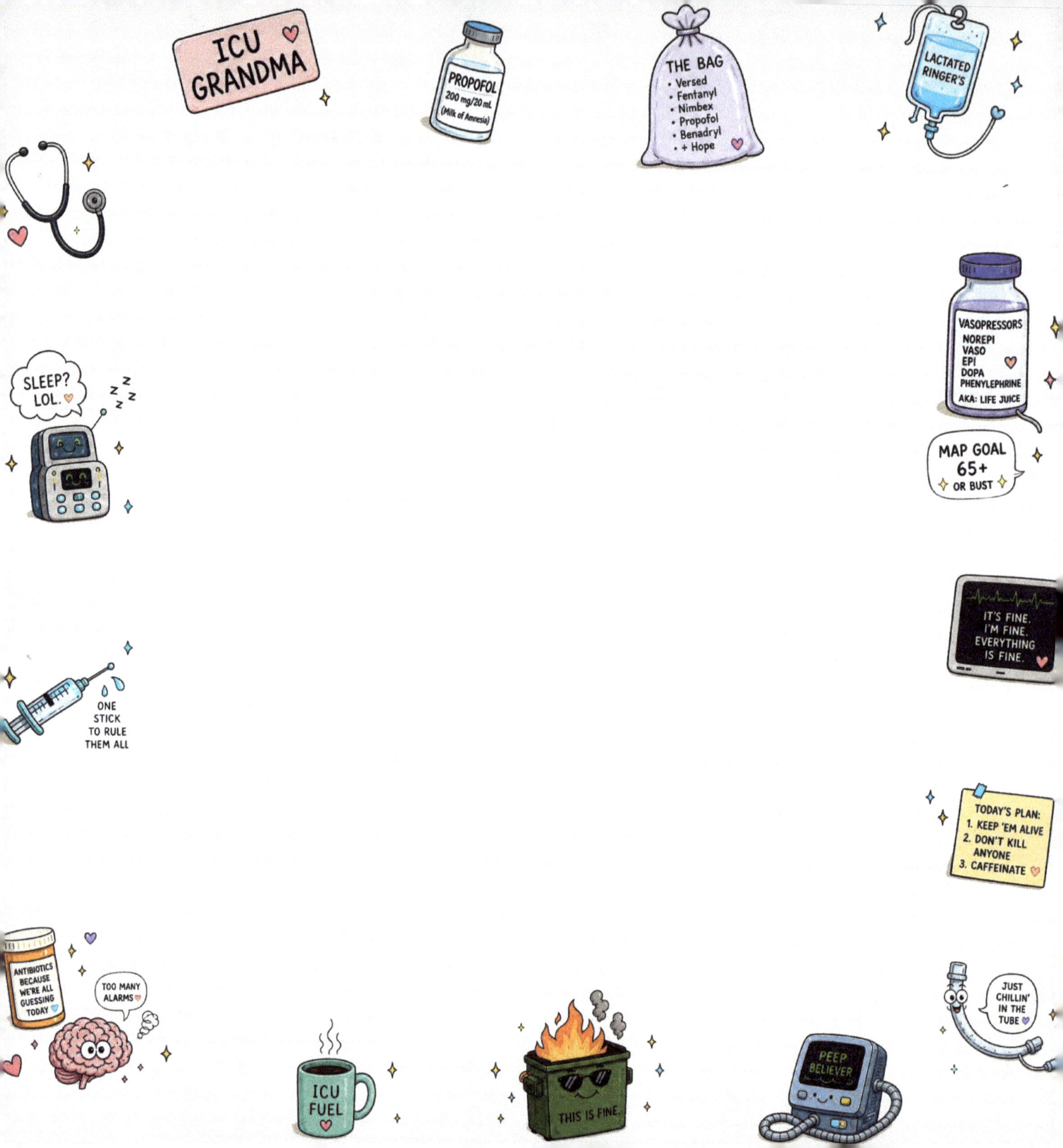
ICU GRANDMA
PROPOFOL 200 mg/20 mL (Milk of Amnesia)
THE BAG
• Versed
• Fentanyl
• Nimbex
• Propofol
• Benadryl
• + Hope
LACTATED RINGER'S
VASOPRESSORS
NOREPI
VASO
EPI
DOPA
PHENYLEPHRINE
AKA: LIFE JUICE
MAP GOAL 65+ OR BUST
SLEEP? LOL.
IT'S FINE. I'M FINE. EVERYTHING IS FINE.
ONE STICK TO RULE THEM ALL
TODAY'S PLAN:
1. KEEP 'EM ALIVE
2. DON'T KILL ANYONE
3. CAFFEINATE
ANTIBIOTICS BECAUSE WE'RE ALL GUESSING TODAY
TOO MANY ALARMS
ICU FUEL
THIS IS FINE.
PEEP BELIEVER
JUST CHILLIN' IN THE TUBE

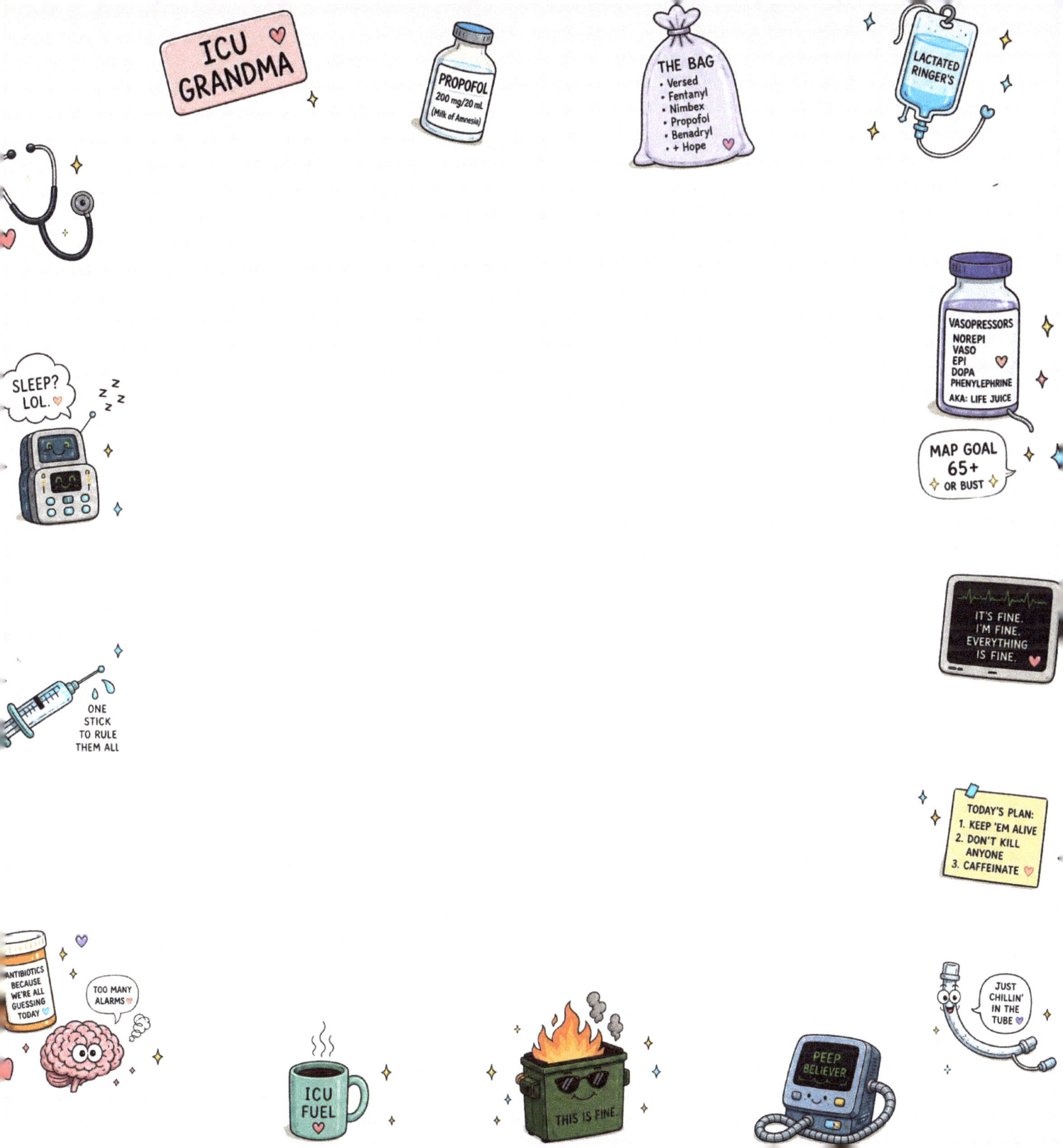
ICU GRANDMA
PROPOFOL
200 mg/20 mL
(Milk of Amnesia)
THE BAG
• Versed
• Fentanyl
• Nimbex
• Propofol
• Benadryl
• + Hope
LACTATED RINGER'S
VASOPRESSORS
NOREPI
VASO
EPI
DOPA
PHENYLEPHRINE
AKA: LIFE JUICE
MAP GOAL 65+ OR BUST
SLEEP? LOL.
IT'S FINE. I'M FINE. EVERYTHING IS FINE.
ONE STICK TO RULE THEM ALL
TODAY'S PLAN:
1. KEEP 'EM ALIVE
2. DON'T KILL ANYONE
3. CAFFEINATE
ANTIBIOTICS BECAUSE WE'RE ALL GUESSING TODAY
TOO MANY ALARMS
ICU FUEL
THIS IS FINE.
PEEP BELIEVER
JUST CHILLIN' IN THE TUBE

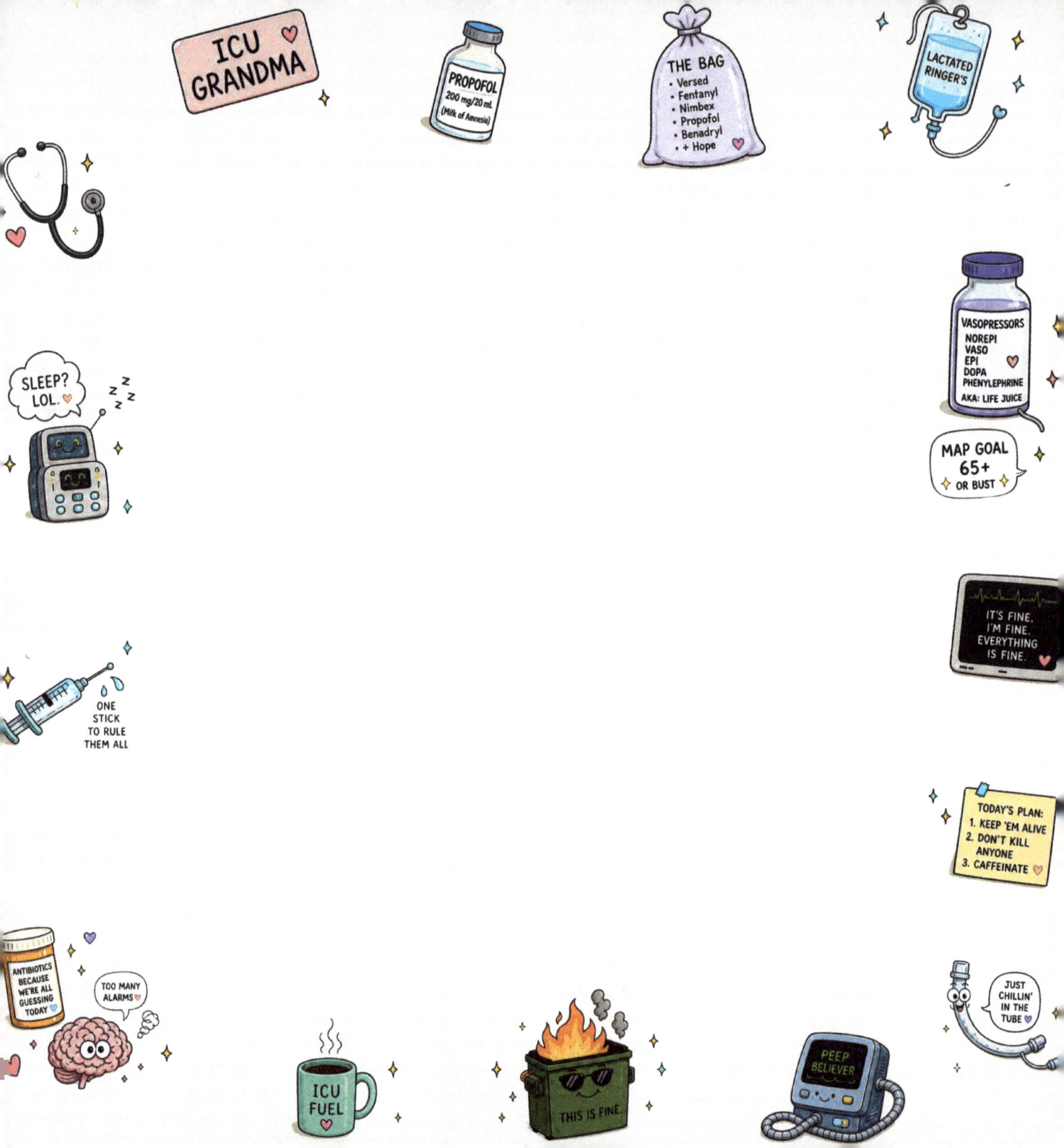
ICU GRANDMA
PROPOFOL
200 mg/20 mL
(Milk of Amnesia)
THE BAG
• Versed
• Fentanyl
• Nimbex
• Propofol
• Benadryl
• + Hope
LACTATED RINGER'S
VASOPRESSORS
NOREPI
VASO
EPI
DOPA
PHENYLEPHRINE
AKA: LIFE JUICE
MAP GOAL
65+
OR BUST
SLEEP? LOL.
Z Z Z Z
IT'S FINE, I'M FINE. EVERYTHING IS FINE.
ONE STICK TO RULE THEM ALL
TODAY'S PLAN:
1. KEEP 'EM ALIVE
2. DON'T KILL ANYONE
3. CAFFEINATE
ANTIBIOTICS BECAUSE WE'RE ALL GUESSING TODAY
TOO MANY ALARMS
ICU FUEL
THIS IS FINE.
PEEP BELIEVER
JUST CHILLIN' IN THE TUBE

www.ingramcontent.com/pod-product-compliance
Lightning Source LLC
LaVergne TN
LVHW070900210926
848482LV00016B/986
9798995907916